ULTIMATE PCOS DIET COOKBOOK FOR WOMEN:

"Healthy and Delicious Recipes for Managing PCOS Symptoms"

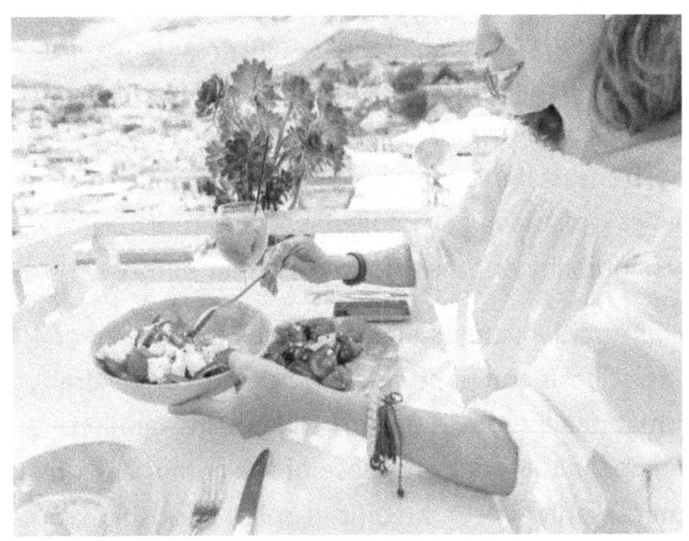

Dr. VERA J. REYNOLD

This book is a work of non-fiction. The information, opinions, and advice presented in this book are based on the author's research and personal experience. The author and publisher make no representation or warranties with respect to the accuracy or completeness of the contents of this book and specifically disclaim any implied warranties of merchantability or fitness for a particular purpose.

The information contained in this book is provided on an "as is" basis and is intended to be used for general informational purposes only. The views and opinions expressed in this book are those of the author and do not necessarily reflect the official policy or position of any agency, organization, employer, or company.

Contents

INTRODUCTION

My aunt, Rachel, had always been health-conscious, so it was a shock when she was diagnosed with Polycystic Ovary Syndrome (PCOS) in her mid-20s. The symptoms began to take a toll on her health - she gained weight, fought with acne, and suffered from irregular periods. Rachel tried every medicine and therapy available, but nothing seemed to help. She was desperate to find a solution to her PCOS symptoms, but it wasn't until she ran into a PCOS diet cookbook that things began to change.

At first, Rachel was suspicious. She had tried numerous diets previously, but nothing alleviated her PCOS problems. However, the more she read about the PCOS diet, the more it made sense. The cookbook stressed the significance of nutrient-dense whole foods and avoiding processed and high-sugar meals, which are known to induce inflammation and worsen PCOS symptoms. The cookbook also stressed balancing macronutrients, including healthy fats, proteins, and carbs, to manage insulin levels and optimize metabolic health.

Rachel decided to try the PCOS diet cookbook, and she never looked back. The cookbook contained a broad selection of tasty and easy-to-prepare PCOS-friendly recipes, including morning smoothies, quinoa bowls, and stir-fry entrees. She realized that she could still eat the foods she liked but in a manner that fed her body and minimized her symptoms.

Within a few weeks of starting the PCOS diet, Rachel noticed significant improvements in her PCOS symptoms. Her energy levels were up, her acne started to clean up, and her periods were more regular. After a few months, she lost weight and felt better than in years.

Rachel's experience with the PCOS diet was life-changing. She learned that she didn't have to depend on medication or therapies to control her symptoms; rather, she could utilize food as medicine. She began educating herself more about nutrition and experimenting with various PCOS-friendly dishes.

Rachel's experience with the PCOS diet encouraged her to assist other women battling the same issue. She launched a blog where she recounted her personal PCOS story and offered PCOS-friendly foods and lifestyle suggestions. She even organized a support group for people with PCOS in her town.

In conclusion, the PCOS diet cookbook helped my aunt Rachel control her PCOS symptoms in a manner that she had never experienced before. The key to her success was the nutrient-dense whole foods, balanced macronutrients, and PCOS-friendly dishes. If you or someone you know is battling with PCOS, consider trying the PCOS diet and see if it will assist you too.

PCOS, or Polycystic Ovary Syndrome, is a hormonal condition that affects up to 10% of women of reproductive age. The symptoms of PCOS may be tough to manage, from weight gain and irregular periods to acne and hair growth. However, studies have shown that changes in diet and lifestyle can help alleviate symptoms and improve overall health outcomes for those with PCOS.

This is where the PCOS diet cookbook comes in. It is a complete book that includes useful advice on how to diet for PCOS, along with tasty and nutritious meals that are particularly created to benefit persons with PCOS. This cookbook is not just a recipe book. Still, it also provides educational information on PCOS, such as understanding the fundamental causes of the illness, recognizing common symptoms, and addressing dietary deficiencies that may worsen PCOS symptoms.

By following the directions and recipes in the PCOS diet cookbook, many women have experienced dramatic changes in their PCOS symptoms, from better management of their menstrual cycles to weight reduction and enhanced fertility. The cookbook's focus on complete, nutrient-dense meals and avoiding inflammatory foods may help lower insulin resistance, balance hormones, and promote gut health.

The PCOS diet cookbook is a fantastic resource that gives practical direction and assistance for anybody battling PCOS symptoms or wanting to enhance their health and fitness. It is a recipe book and a thorough handbook that enables women to take charge of their health via good diet and self-care.

CHAPTER ONE

What is PCOS?

PCOS stands for Polycystic Ovary Syndrome. It is a hormonal condition that affects reproductive-aged women. Women with PCOS have uneven levels of hormones, which may cause several symptoms, including irregular periods, increased hair growth, weight gain, acne, and infertility. PCOS is also related to an increased risk of various health conditions such as type 2 diabetes, high blood pressure, and cardiovascular disease. The specific etiology of PCOS is not entirely known. However, it is likely associated with hereditary and environmental factors. Diagnosis of PCOS often requires a physical exam, blood testing, and ultrasound imaging of the ovaries. Treatment may entail lifestyle modifications such as nutrition and exercise, medication to control menstrual periods or insulin levels, and even surgery.

How might food help control PCOS?

Diet may play an essential part in controlling PCOS. Women with PCOS commonly develop insulin resistance, which means their bodies have problems utilizing insulin adequately. Insulin is a hormone that helps control blood sugar levels, and when it is not utilized efficiently, it may contribute to weight gain, a higher risk of type 2 diabetes, and other health concerns. Research has indicated that dietary adjustments may help increase insulin sensitivity and control PCOS symptoms.

Some dietary advice for controlling PCOS includes:

1. **Choosing complex carbohydrates:** Foods high in fiber and complex carbohydrates, such as whole grains, fruits, and vegetables, can help regulate blood sugar levels and improve insulin sensitivity.

2. **Eating lean protein:** Choosing lean protein sources such as fish, chicken, turkey, and lentils may help regulate blood sugar levels and promote good weight control.

3. **Including healthy fats:** Incorporating healthy fats such as those found in nuts, seeds, and avocados can help reduce inflammation and support hormonal balance.

4. **Avoiding processed and sugary foods:** Processed foods and those rich in added sugars may contribute to rises in blood sugar levels and aggravate insulin resistance.

5. **Maintaining a healthy weight:** For women with PCOS who are overweight or obese, decreasing weight via diet and exercise may help improve insulin sensitivity and lessen symptoms.

Engaging with a healthcare practitioner or registered dietitian is crucial to building a specific dietary plan for treating PCOS.

Overview of the PCOS Cookbook

The PCOS Cookbook is a resource for people with Polycystic Ovary Syndrome (PCOS) who are hoping to treat their symptoms via dietary modifications. The cookbook contains a range of dishes that are aimed to be low in processed carbs and sweets and rich in fiber, healthy fats, and lean protein. The recipes are centered on complete, nutrient-dense meals and offer alternatives for breakfast, lunch, supper, snacks, and desserts.

In addition to recipes, the cookbook also contains information about the significance of nutrition in controlling PCOS, recommendations for stocking a PCOS-friendly kitchen, and example meal plans. The cookbook highlights the necessity of a balanced and diverse diet and includes suggestions on integrating nutrient-rich foods that may help control PCOS symptoms.

Overall, the PCOS Cookbook is a comprehensive resource that gives practical direction and support for women with PCOS trying to make dietary adjustments to enhance their health and well-being.

CHAPTER TWO

Understanding PCOS and Nutrition

Understanding PCOS

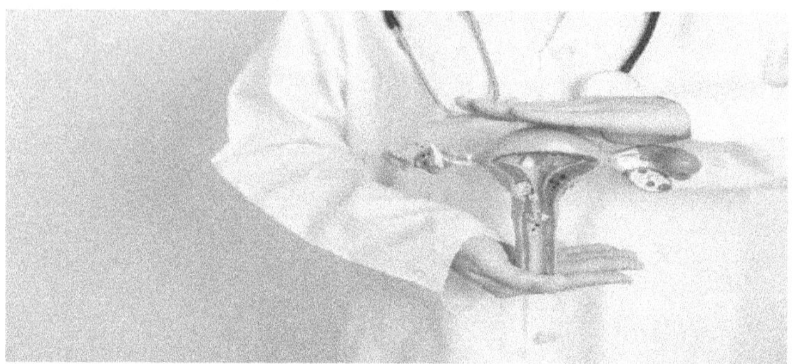

Polycystic Ovary Syndrome (PCOS) is a hormonal condition that affects women of reproductive age. PCOS is characterized by uneven amounts of several hormones, particularly increased levels of androgens (male hormones) and insulin. This hormonal imbalance may lead to a range of symptoms, including:

1. **Irregular menstrual periods:** Women with PCOS may suffer infrequent, irregular, or extended periods.

2. **Excess hair growth:** Due to the high amounts of androgens, women with PCOS may suffer excess hair growth on their face, chest, back, or stomach.

3. **Acne:** Elevated androgen levels may also contribute to acne or greasy skin.

4. **Weight increase:** Many women with PCOS battle with weight gain, especially in the stomach region.

5. **Infertility:** PCOS is a prevalent cause of infertility owing to irregular menstrual cycles and issues with ovulation.

6. **Other health concerns:** Women with PCOS are at higher risk of developing other health issues such as type 2 diabetes, high blood pressure, and cardiovascular disease.

The specific etiology of PCOS is not entirely known. However, it is likely associated with hereditary and environmental factors. There is no cure for PCOS, but the symptoms may be treated with lifestyle modifications, medicine, and other therapies. Women with PCOS must collaborate with their physicians to build an individualized treatment plan that addresses their unique symptoms and concerns.

Symptoms and diagnosis

The symptoms of PCOS may vary from person to person, and not all women with PCOS will experience all of the symptoms. The most prevalent symptoms include:

1. **Irregular periods:** Women with PCOS may have fewer than eight periods per year or may suffer heavy, protracted, or unexpected periods.

2. **Excess hair growth:** Elevated levels of androgens may produce excess hair growth on the face, chest, back, or stomach.

3. **Acne:** Increased androgen levels may also contribute to acne or greasy skin.

4. **Weight increase:** Many women with PCOS battle with weight gain, especially in the stomach region.

5. **Infertility:** PCOS is a prevalent cause of infertility owing to irregular menstrual cycles and issues with ovulation.

6. **Other health concerns:** Women with PCOS are at higher risk of developing other health issues such as type 2 diabetes, high blood pressure, and cardiovascular disease.

To diagnose PCOS, a healthcare professional would often do a physical exam and inquire about the patient's medical history and symptoms. They may also request blood tests to monitor hormone levels and an ultrasound to search for cysts on the ovaries. To be diagnosed with PCOS, a woman must have at least two out of three of the following criteria:

1. Irregular periods or no periods at all.

2. Elevated amounts of androgens, as revealed by blood testing.

3. Cysts on the ovaries, as discovered by ultrasonography.

It's crucial to note that some women with PCOS may have ovaries that do not have cysts and that a diagnosis of PCOS may only be determined by a healthcare specialist following a complete assessment.

Causes and risk factors

The specific origin of PCOS is not entirely known, although research shows that both hereditary and environmental factors may play a role. Some of the recognized risk factors and suspected causes of PCOS include:

1. **Insulin resistance:** Many women with PCOS have insulin resistance, which means their body's cells are less receptive to insulin, a hormone that helps control blood sugar levels. This may induce the pancreas to generate more insulin, which can increase testosterone production and interrupt ovulation.

2. **Genetics:** PCOS tends to run in families, indicating that there may be a hereditary component to the illness.

3. **Inflammation:** Chronic inflammation may have a role in developing PCOS since it may contribute to insulin resistance and high testosterone levels.

4. **Lifestyle factors:** Obesity, a sedentary lifestyle, and a diet heavy in refined carbs and sweets may raise the chance of developing PCOS.

5. **Hormonal imbalances:** PCOS is characterized by abnormalities in levels of several hormones, including androgens, insulin, and luteinizing hormone (LH).

6. **Environmental factors:** Exposure to endocrine-disrupting chemicals (EDCs) such as BPA,

phthalates, and dioxins may contribute to the development of PCOS.

It's essential to note that although these characteristics may raise the likelihood of having PCOS, not all women with these risk factors will acquire the illness. Some women without these risk factors may still develop PCOS. The actual etiology of PCOS is complicated and may entail a mix of several variables.

Nutrition and PCOS

Nutrition has a significant part in treating PCOS symptoms. Women with PCOS may benefit from a balanced diet with various nutrient-rich foods. Here are some nutrition-related tips that may help manage PCOS:

1. **Focus on fiber:** Eating a diet high in fiber may help manage blood sugar levels and reduce insulin resistance. Choose whole grains, fruits, veggies, and legumes to enhance your fiber intake.

2. **Choose good fats:** Consuming healthy fats, such as those found in nuts, seeds, avocados, and fatty fish, may help decrease inflammation and enhance hormonal balance.

3. **Limit refined carbs:** Refined carbohydrates, such as those in sugary beverages, white bread, and

pastries, may induce blood sugar surges and aggravate insulin resistance.

4. **Eat protein at every meal:** Protein may help manage blood sugar levels and keep you feeling full. Choose lean protein sources such as chicken, turkey, fish, tofu, and lentils.

5. **Balance your meals:** Aim to incorporate a mix of complex carbs, healthy fats, and protein in each meal to help balance blood sugar levels and prevent insulin resistance.

6. **Consider supplements:** Certain supplements, such as inositol, may help improve insulin sensitivity and hormone balance in women with PCOS. Talk to your healthcare physician before taking any supplements.

It's crucial to realize that every woman with PCOS is unique and may have distinct dietary demands. Working with a registered dietitian or healthcare practitioner may help you establish a tailored nutrition plan that suits your particular requirements and objectives.

How diet affects PCOS

Diet may have a big influence on PCOS symptoms. Eating a balanced and nutrient-dense diet may help improve insulin resistance, decrease inflammation, and regulate hormone levels, all of which are essential variables in controlling PCOS symptoms. Here are some specific ways that diet can affect PCOS:

1. **Insulin resistance:** Women with PCOS are at higher risk of insulin resistance, which may lead to high blood sugar levels, weight gain, and increased androgen production. A strong diet of refined carbs and sweets might cause insulin resistance. In contrast, a balanced diet that contains complex carbs, fiber, healthy fats, and protein may help manage blood sugar levels and enhance insulin sensitivity.

2. **Hormonal balance:** PCOS is characterized by abnormalities in levels of several hormones, including androgens, insulin, and luteinizing hormone (LH). A diet that is low in nutrient-dense meals and heavy in processed and inflammatory foods may lead to hormone abnormalities. Eating a balanced and nutrient-dense diet may help regulate hormone levels and minimize symptoms such as acne, increased hair growth, and irregular periods.

3. **Inflammation:** Chronic inflammation is likely to have a role in developing PCOS since it may lead to insulin resistance and hormonal abnormalities. Eating a diet heavy in anti-inflammatory foods, such as fruits, vegetables, whole grains, and fatty fish, may help decrease inflammation and alleviate PCOS symptoms.

Overall, a balanced and nutrient-dense diet that includes a range of whole foods may help treat PCOS symptoms by lowering insulin resistance, regulating hormone levels, and reducing inflammation. Working with a registered dietitian or healthcare practitioner may help you establish a tailored nutrition plan that suits your particular requirements and objectives.

Nutritional deficits and PCOS

Women with PCOS may be at higher risk of various nutritional deficiencies for several reasons, including dietary preferences, insulin resistance, and hormonal abnormalities. Here are some common nutritional deficiencies that may occur in women with PCOS:

1. **Vitamin D:** Vitamin D insufficiency is frequent in women with PCOS and may be associated with insulin resistance and other PCOS-related symptoms such as irregular periods and infertility. Adequate vitamin D consumption is necessary for

bone health, immunological function, and hormonal balance.

2. **Magnesium:** Magnesium is necessary for insulin sensitivity and glucose control. Magnesium insufficiency has been connected with insulin resistance and metabolic syndrome, both frequent in women with PCOS.

3. **Zinc:** is crucial for immune function, wound healing, and reproductive health. Women with PCOS may have reduced amounts of zinc, which may alter hormonal balance and lead to inflammation.

4. **Omega-3 fatty acids:** Omega-3 fatty acids, found in fatty fish, flaxseeds, and chia seeds, have anti-inflammatory qualities and may help regulate menstrual cycles in people with PCOS.

5. **B vitamins:** B vitamins are necessary for energy generation and hormonal homeostasis. Women with PCOS may have reduced amounts of various B vitamins, particularly folate and vitamin B12.

6. **Iron:** Women with heavy or irregular periods may be at higher risk of iron deficiency anemia. Iron is crucial for energy synthesis, immunological function, and oxygen transfer.

It's vital for women with PCOS to obtain frequent blood testing to check for any nutritional deficits. Working with a qualified dietitian or healthcare practitioner may help you establish a tailored nutrition plan that suits your particular requirements and treats any nutritional deficits. In certain circumstances, supplements may be advised to treat particular deficiencies.

Common dietary advice for PCOS

Here are some common dietary recommendations for women with PCOS:

1. **Focus on nutrient-dense whole foods:** Eating a range of nutrients, including fruits, vegetables, whole grains, lean protein, and healthy fats, will help manage blood sugar levels, increase insulin sensitivity, and decrease inflammation.

2. **Choose complex carbs:** Complex carbohydrates, such as whole grains, vegetables, and legumes, are fiber-rich and may help manage blood sugar levels. In contrast, simple carbs, such as white bread, sugary beverages, and processed snacks, may increase blood sugar surges and aggravate insulin resistance.

3. **Include lean protein:** Lean protein sources, such as chicken, fish, tofu, and lentils, may help manage blood sugar levels, decrease inflammation, and enhance satiety.

4. **Incorporate healthy fats:** Healthy fats, such as avocados, nuts, seeds, and olive oil, can help regulate hormones, reduce inflammation, and improve insulin sensitivity.

5. **Limit refined sugars and processed meals:** Refined sugars and processed foods may lead to inflammation, increase insulin resistance, and alter hormonal balance.

6. **Manage portion sizes:** Eating balanced meals with proper portion sizes will help regulate blood sugar levels and assist weight management.

7. **Stay hydrated:** Drinking plenty of water and avoiding sugary drinks can help regulate blood sugar levels and improve overall health.

8. **Consider supplements:** In certain circumstances, vitamin D, magnesium, and omega-3 fatty acids may be advised to treat particular dietary shortages and alleviate PCOS symptoms.

It's crucial to remember that every individual is unique, and dietary advice may vary based on personal tastes, nutritional requirements, and PCOS symptoms. Working with a registered dietitian or healthcare practitioner may help you establish a tailored nutrition plan that suits your particular requirements and objectives.

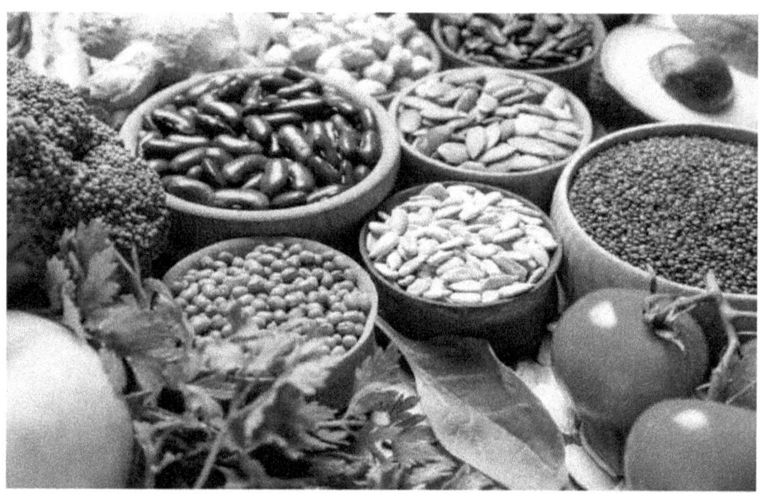

CHAPTER THREE

Breakfast Recipes

Greek yogurt with berries and nuts/seeds

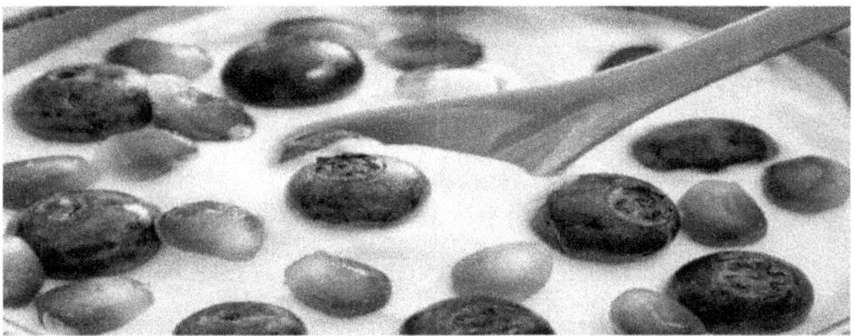

Greek yogurt with berries and nuts/seeds is a simple and healthy PCOS-friendly breakfast choice that may help manage blood sugar levels and increase fullness. Here's how to create it:

Ingredients:

- 1 cup of Greek yogurt
- ½ cup of mixed berries (such as blueberries, raspberries, and strawberries)
- Two tablespoons of chopped nuts and/or seeds (such as almonds, walnuts, or chia seeds)
- **Optional:** sprinkle honey or maple syrup for sweetness

Instructions:

1. Spoon the Greek yogurt into a bowl.
2. Rinse the berries and place them on top of the yogurt.
3. Chop the nuts and seeds and sprinkle them on top of the berries.
4. Drizzle with honey or maple syrup if preferred.

You may also vary the berries and nuts/seeds to make new taste combinations or add a sprinkle of cinnamon or vanilla essence for added flavor. This meal is strong in protein, fiber, and healthy fats, which may help keep you full and satisfied throughout the morning.

Veggie omelet

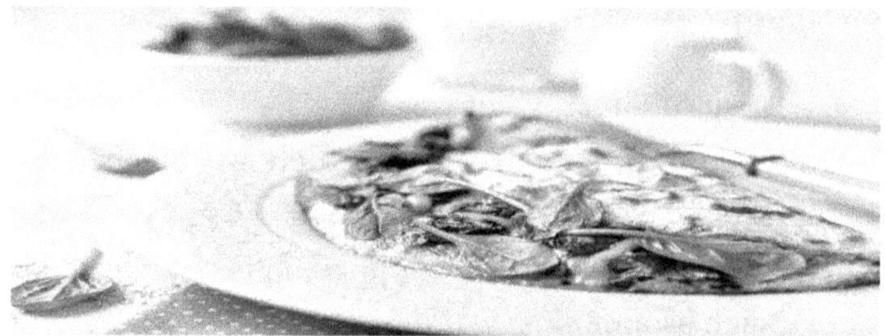

A vegetarian omelet is a tasty and nutritious PCOS-friendly breakfast choice that is strong in protein, fiber, and healthy fats. Here's how to create it:

Ingredients:

- Two eggs
- 1/2 cup of chopped veggies (such as spinach, mushrooms, bell peppers, onions, or broccoli)
- 1/4 avocado or ¼ cup of shredded cheese
- One tablespoon of olive oil or coconut oil
- Salt and pepper to taste

Instructions:

1. Heat a non-stick pan over medium-high heat and add the oil.
2. Add the chopped veggies to the pan and sauté for a few minutes until soft.

3. Beat the eggs in a basin and pour them over the veggies.

4. Use a spatula to carefully raise the edges of the omelet and allow the raw eggs to pour below.

5. Add the avocado or shredded cheese on one side of the omelet when the eggs are nearly set.

6. Use the spatula to fold the opposite side of the omelet over the filling.

7. Cook for a further minute until the cheese is melted or the avocado is heated.

8. Season with salt and pepper to taste.

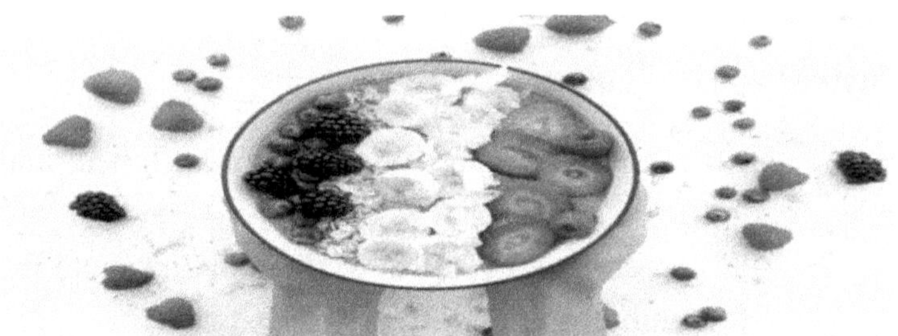

A smoothie bowl is a pleasant, nutrient-dense, PCOS-friendly breakfast option full of fiber, vitamins, and minerals. Here's how to create it:

Ingredients:

- One frozen banana
- 1 cup of frozen mixed berries (such as blueberries, raspberries, and strawberries)
- ½ cup of spinach or kale leaves
- ½ cup of unsweetened almond milk or coconut milk
- One spoonful of chia seeds or flax seeds
- **Toppings:** sliced fruits, chopped nuts, coconut flakes, or granola

Instructions:

1. Add the frozen banana, mixed berries, spinach or kale leaves, almond or coconut milk, and chia or flax seeds to a blender.

2. Blend until smooth and creamy.

3. Pour the smoothie into a bowl.

4. Top with sliced fruits, chopped nuts, coconut flakes, or granola.

Quinoa breakfast bowl

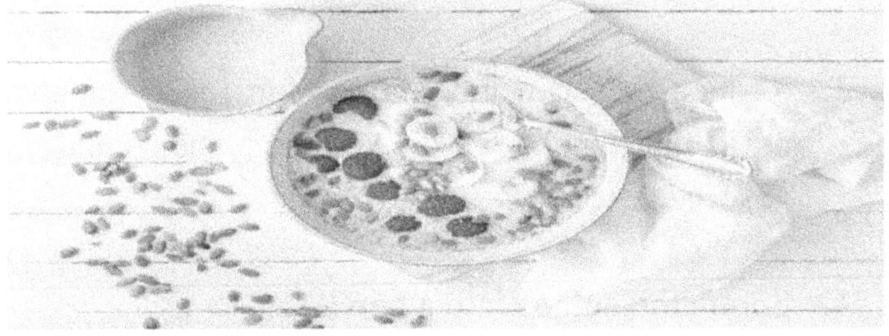

A quinoa breakfast bowl is a robust and nutritious PCOS-friendly breakfast option full of protein, fiber, and complex carbs. Here's how to create it:

Ingredients:

- ½ cup of quinoa

- 1 cup of unsweetened almond milk or coconut milk
- ½ teaspoon of ground cinnamon
- ½ cup of mixed berries (such as blueberries, raspberries, and strawberries)
- ¼ cup of chopped nuts (such as almonds, walnuts, or pecans)
- **Optional:** sprinkle honey or maple syrup for sweetness

Instructions:

1. Rinse the quinoa under cold water and drain.

2. Add the quinoa, almond milk or coconut milk, and cinnamon to a saucepan and boil.

3. Reduce the heat and simmer for 15-20 minutes until the quinoa is cooked and the liquid is absorbed.

4. Spoon the quinoa into a bowl.

5. Top with mixed berries and chopped nuts.

6. Drizzle with honey or maple syrup if preferred.

7. Serve and enjoy!

Add a dollop of Greek yogurt or a sprinkle of coconut flakes for added creaminess and flavor. This breakfast bowl is a terrific way to integrate nutritious grains, fruits, and nuts into your daily routine, which may help balance blood sugar levels and give sustained energy throughout the day.

Chia seed pudding

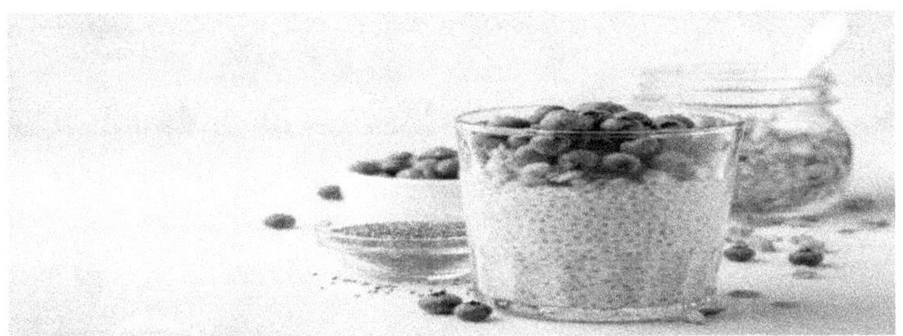

Chia seed pudding is a simple and tasty PCOS-friendly breakfast option packed with fiber, healthy fats, and antioxidants. Here's how to create it:

Ingredients:

- ¼ cup of chia seeds
- 1 cup of unsweetened almond milk or coconut milk
- ½ teaspoon of vanilla extract
- **Optional:** sprinkle honey or maple syrup for sweetness
- **Toppings:** sliced fruits, chopped nuts, coconut flakes, or granola

Instructions:

1. Blend the chia seeds, almond milk or coconut milk, and vanilla essence in a bowl.

2. Whisk the ingredients until fully mixed.

3. Let the mixture settle for 5 minutes, then whisk again.

4. Cover the bowl and refrigerate for at least 2 hours or overnight.

5. Once the pudding has thickened, could you give it a good stir?

6. Spoon the pudding into a bowl.

7. Top with sliced fruits, chopped nuts, coconut flakes, or granola.

8. Drizzle with honey or maple syrup if preferred.

You may also experiment with other tastes by adding cocoa powder, cinnamon, or match powder to the pudding recipe. This chia seed pudding is a terrific way to start your day with a healthy and enjoyable meal that may help manage blood sugar levels and support hormonal balance.

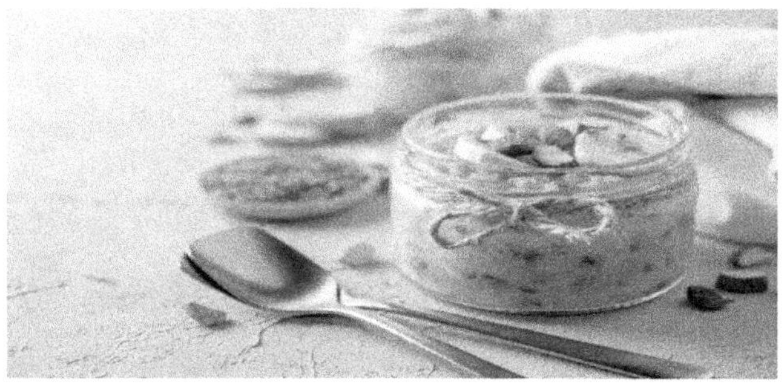

Ingredients:

- ½ cup of rolled oats
- ½ cup of unsweetened almond milk or coconut milk
- ½ teaspoon of vanilla extract
- One tablespoon of chia seeds
- **Optional:** sprinkle honey or maple syrup for sweetness
- **Toppings:** sliced fruits, chopped nuts, coconut flakes, or granola

Instructions:

1. Mix the rolled oats, almond milk or coconut milk, vanilla essence, and chia seeds in a jar or container with a cover.

2. Stir well to mix.

3. Cover the jar or container with a cover and refrigerate overnight or for at least 4 hours.

4. Once the oats have absorbed the liquid and become thick and creamy, could you stir it?

5. Top with sliced fruits, chopped nuts, coconut flakes, or granola.

6. Drizzle with honey or maple syrup if preferred.

You may also add a scoop of protein powder, nut butter, or Greek yogurt to the oats for more protein and creaminess. Overnight oats are a terrific way to save time in the morning and still have a healthy and satisfying meal that may help manage blood sugar levels and support hormonal balance.

Breakfast smoothies and bowls

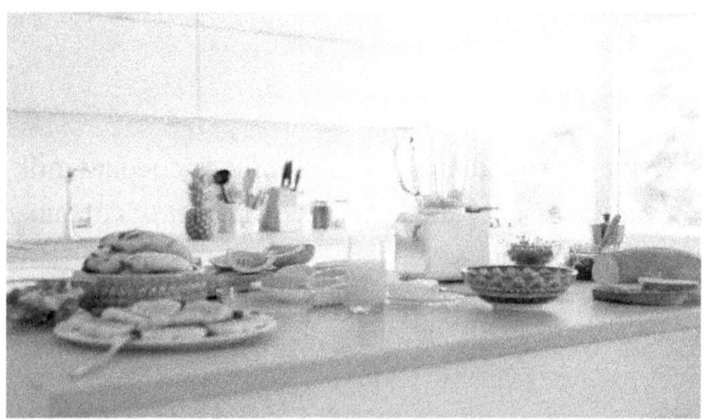

Smoothies and bowls are a terrific way to cram a variety of nutrients into your morning. Here are some PCOS-friendly breakfast smoothie and bowl ideas:

1. **Green smoothie:** In a blender, combine 1 cup of unsweetened almond milk, 1 cup of spinach or kale, 1/2 cup of frozen berries, 1/2 banana, one tablespoon of chia seeds, and one scoop of protein powder.
   Optional: add a drizzle of honey or maple syrup for sweetness.

2. **Berry smoothie bowl:** In a blender, combine 1 cup of unsweetened almond milk, 1 cup of frozen berries, 1/2 banana, one tablespoon of chia seeds, and one scoop of protein powder. Pour the smoothie into a bowl and top with sliced fruits, chopped nuts, coconut flakes, or granola.

3. **Chocolate protein smoothie:** In a blender, combine 1 cup of unsweetened almond milk, one scoop of chocolate protein powder, one spoonful of almond butter, 1/2 banana, and a handful of ice cubes. Optional: add a drizzle of honey or maple syrup for sweetness.

4. **Acai bowl:** In a blender, combine one pack of frozen acai puree, 1/2 banana, 1/4 cup of unsweetened almond milk, and one scoop of protein powder. Pour the mixture into a bowl and

top with sliced fruits, chopped nuts, coconut flakes, or granola.

5. **Yogurt smoothie:** In a blender, combine 1 cup of Greek yogurt, 1/2 cup of frozen berries, 1/2 banana, one tablespoon of chia seeds, and a handful of ice cubes. Optional: add a drizzle of honey or maple syrup for sweetness.

Smoothies and bowls are adaptable and may be readily adjusted to meet your taste preferences and nutritional concerns. They may contain some nutrients that can help regulate PCOS symptoms, including fiber, healthy fats, protein, and antioxidants.

Breakfast sandwiches and wraps

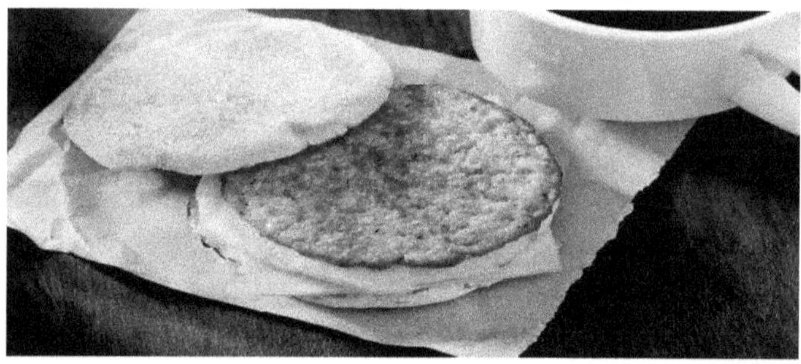

Here are some PCOS-friendly breakfast sandwich and wrap ideas:

1. **Egg and avocado sandwich:** Toast whole grain bread and put mashed avocado on top. Top with a fried or scrambled egg and a sprinkling of salt and

pepper. Optional: add sliced tomato or spinach for added nutrition.

2. **Breakfast burrito:** Scramble eggs with chopped bell peppers and onions, then add a teaspoon of black beans. Wrap the mixture in a whole-grain tortilla, then top with salsa or guacamole.

3. **Greek yogurt and berry wrap:** Spread Greek yogurt over a whole grain tortilla, then top with mixed berries and a sprinkling of cinnamon. Roll up the tortilla and enjoy.

4. **Smoked salmon bagel sandwich:** Toast a whole-grain bagel, then put a layer of cream cheese on each side. Top with sliced smoked salmon, red onion, and capers.

5. **Veggie and hummus wrap:** Spread hummus on a whole grain tortilla, then add sliced cucumber, carrot, and bell pepper. Roll up the tortilla and enjoy.

These breakfast sandwiches and wraps are simple to create and may give a balanced blend of protein, healthy fats, and carbs. They may also be customized with various fillings and toppings to suit your taste preferences and dietary concerns.

CHAPTER FOUR

Lunch Recipes

Quinoa and roasted veggie salad

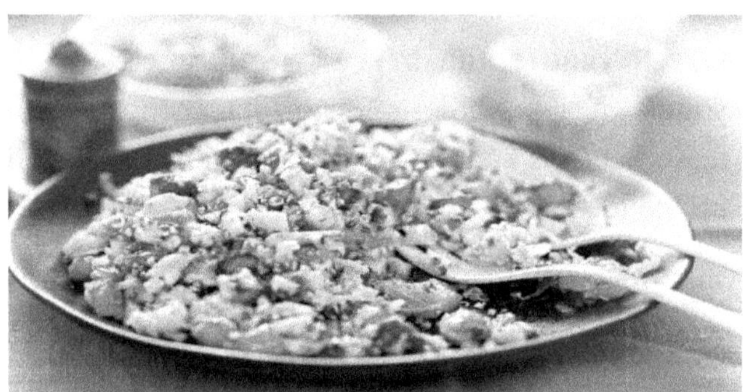

Ingredients:

- 1 cup quinoa
- 2 cups water or vegetable broth
- One red bell pepper, chopped
- One zucchini, diced one red onion, diced two tablespoons olive oil
- Salt and pepper to taste
- 2 cups baby spinach or arugula
- Two tablespoons of balsamic vinegar

Instructions:

1. Preheat the oven to 400°F.

2. Rinse the quinoa in cool water and drain. Add the quinoa, water, or vegetable broth to a saucepan, and boil. Reduce heat to low, cover, and simmer for 15-20 minutes or until the quinoa is cooked and the water is absorbed.

3. While the quinoa is cooking, toss the diced bell pepper, zucchini, and red onion with olive oil, salt, and pepper. Spread the veggies on a baking sheet in a single layer and roast in the oven for 20-25 minutes or until the vegetables are soft and slightly browned.

4. Combine the cooked quinoa with the roasted veggies in a large mixing dish. Add the baby spinach or arugula, and mix to incorporate.

5. Drizzle the balsamic vinegar over the salad, and toss to coat.

6. Serve warm or cold.

This salad is a tasty and healthful way to integrate quinoa and roasted veggies into your diet. It's packed with fiber, protein, and vitamins and may offer a filling supper that can help control PCOS symptoms.

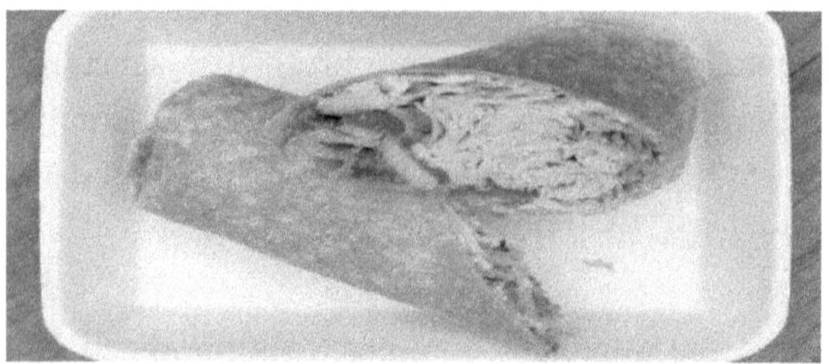

Ingredients:

- Four big lettuce leaves, such as romaine or butter lettuce
- Eight oz. turkey breast, sliced one avocado, mashed one small tomato, diced 1/2 cucumber, sliced
- Salt and pepper to taste

Instructions:

1. Rinse the lettuce leaves and pat dry. Lay the lettuce leaves on a flat surface.

2. Spread 1-2 teaspoons of mashed avocado on each lettuce leaf.

3. Add two oz. Of sliced turkey breast to each lettuce leaf, followed by chopped tomato and sliced cucumber.

4. Sprinkle it with salt & pepper to taste.

5. Roll up the lettuce leaf, then fasten it with a toothpick.

This meal is a fast and simple lunch alternative that is low-carb, high-protein, and filled with healthy fats from the avocado. It may help control PCOS symptoms and keep you full and content throughout the day. You may also modify the filling to your desire by adding or swapping items like chopped bell pepper, shredded carrots, or hummus.

Grilled chicken and veggie skewers

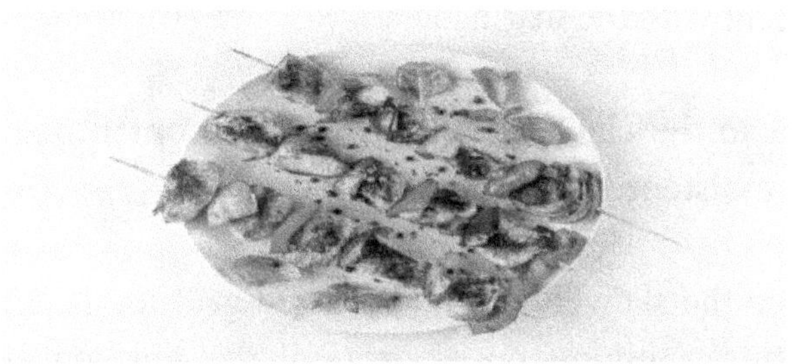

Ingredients:

- One l boneless, skinless chicken breasts cut into 1-inch cubes
- Two bell peppers, seeded and sliced into 1-inch pieces
- One red onion, sliced into 1-inch chunks
- 8-10 wooden skewers soaked in water for at least 30 minutes
- 2 tbsp. olive oil

- 1 tbsp. lemon juice
- Two garlic cloves minced
- Salt and pepper to taste

Instructions:

1. Preheat the grill to medium-high heat.

2. Whisk together the olive oil, lemon juice, garlic, salt, and pepper in a mixing bowl.

3. Add the chicken cubes to the mixing dish, and toss to coat with the marinade.

4. Thread the chicken, bell pepper, and onion onto the moistened wooden skewers.

5. Place the skewers on the prepared grill for 10-12 minutes, turning once, or until the chicken is cooked and the veggies are soft and slightly browned.

This dish is a healthy and tasty way to integrate lean protein and colorful veggies into your diet. It's packed with fiber, vitamins, and minerals and may offer a filling supper that can help control PCOS symptoms. You may also personalize the marinade to your preference by adding herbs or spices like paprika or cumin.

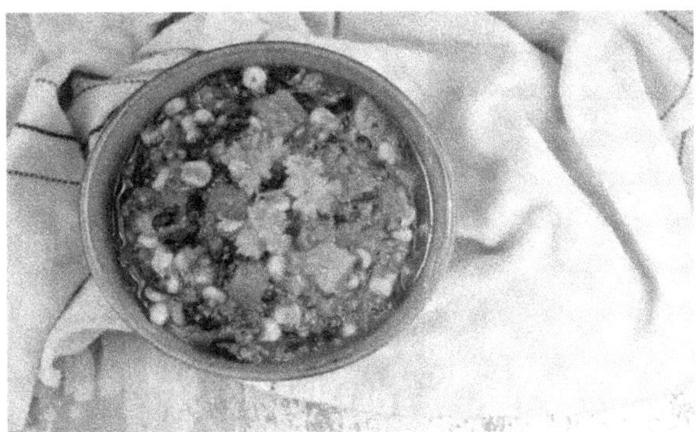

Ingredients:

- Two medium sweet potatoes peeled and cubed
- One can (15 oz.) of black beans, drained and rinsed
- One can (14.5 oz.) diced tomatoes, one undrained onion, two chopped garlic cloves, and minced
- 2 tbsp. olive oil
- 2 tbsp. chili powder
- 1 tsp. ground cumin
- ½ tsp. smoked paprika
- Salt and pepper to taste
- 2 cups vegetable broth

Instructions:

1. In a large saucepan, heat the olive oil over medium heat.

2. Add the chopped onion, minced garlic, and sauté until the onion is transparent for approximately 3-4 minutes.

3. Add the sweet potato cubes, chili powder, ground cumin, smoked paprika, salt, and pepper, and toss to coat.

4. Add the canned black beans and chopped tomatoes (undrained) and mix to incorporate.

5. Pour in the vegetable broth, and bring the mixture to a boil.

6. Reduce the heat to low, cover the saucepan, and simmer for 20-25 minutes or until the sweet potatoes are cooked.

This meal is a substantial and savory vegetarian choice that's high in fiber, protein, and vitamins. Sweet potatoes contain complex carbs that may help manage blood sugar levels, while black beans are a healthy source of plant-based protein and iron. You may alter the recipe by adding or swapping corn, bell peppers, or quinoa.

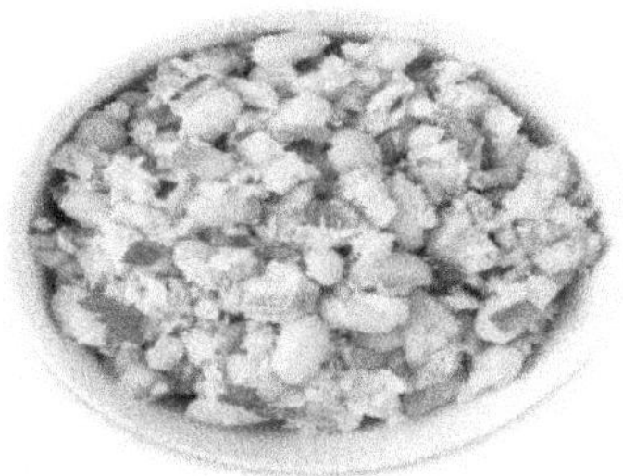

Ingredients:

- Two cans (5 oz. each) of tuna, drained.
- One can (15 oz.) white beans, drained and rinsed ½ red onion, coarsely chopped
- ½ cup cherry tomatoes, halved 1/4 cup Kalamata olives, pitted and chopped
- 2 tbsp. capers
- ¼ cup chopped fresh parsley
- 2 tbsp. olive oil
- 1 tbsp. red wine vinegar
- Salt and pepper to taste

Instructions:

1. Add the drained tuna, white beans, sliced red onion, cherry tomatoes, Kalamata olives, capers, and chopped parsley in a mixing bowl.

2. Mix the olive oil, red wine vinegar, salt, and pepper in a separate bowl.

3. Pour the dressing over the tuna and bean mixture, and toss to coat evenly.

4. Serve cold, and enjoy!

This meal is a nutritious and fulfilling alternative for lunch that's high in protein, fiber, and healthy fats. Tuna is a fantastic source of omega-3 fatty acids, which may help decrease inflammation and improve insulin sensitivity. White beans are a wonderful source of fiber and minerals, while fresh veggies and herbs supply vitamins and antioxidants. You may also tweak the flavor and add extra veggies to your desire.

Lunch bowls and wraps

Here are two recipes for salad bowls and wraps that are PCOS-friendly:

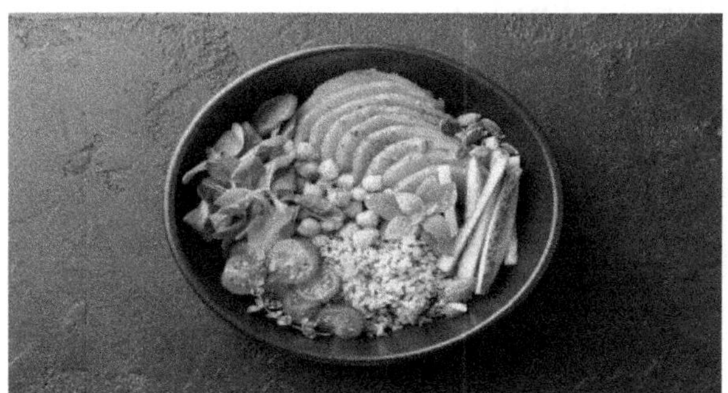

Ingredients:

- 1 cup cooked quinoa
- One can (15 oz.) of chickpeas, drained and rinsed
- ½ cucumber, diced
- ½ red onion, coarsely chopped
- ¼ cup chopped fresh parsley
- 2 tbsp. olive oil
- 1 tbsp. lemon juice
- Salt and pepper to taste

Instructions:

1. Add the cooked quinoa, chickpeas, sliced cucumber, chopped red onion, and fresh parsley in a mixing bowl.

2. Mix the olive oil, lemon juice, salt, and pepper in a separate bowl.

3. Pour the dressing over the quinoa and chickpea mixture, and toss to coat evenly.

4. Serve in a dish or wrap in a lettuce leaf, and enjoy!

This dish is a terrific alternative for a light, refreshing supper packed with protein and fiber. Quinoa and chickpeas are good plant-based protein sources, while cucumber and parsley give vitamins and antioxidants. You may add veggies or toppings, such as chopped tomatoes or sliced avocado.

Turkey and Hummus Wrap

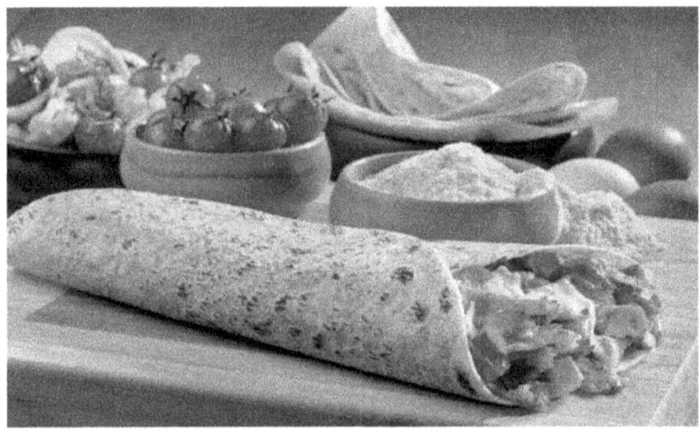

Ingredients:

- One big whole-wheat tortilla
- 4 ounces. sliced turkey breast
- 2 tbsp. hummus
- ½ cucumber, cut ½ red bell pepper, sliced
- ¼ cup baby spinach leaves

Instructions:

1. Spread the hummus over the whole wheat tortilla.

2. Layer the sliced turkey breast, cucumber, red bell pepper, and baby spinach leaves over the hummus.

3. Roll up the tortilla securely, and cut it in half.

4. Serve immediately and enjoy!

This meal is a tasty and hearty alternative that's low in carbs and strong in protein. The turkey breast delivers lean protein, while the hummus adds healthful fats and taste. The veggies offer crunch, fiber, and vitamins. You may also swap various meats or veggies according to your tastes.

Lunch Soups and stews

Creamy Broccoli Soup

Ingredients:

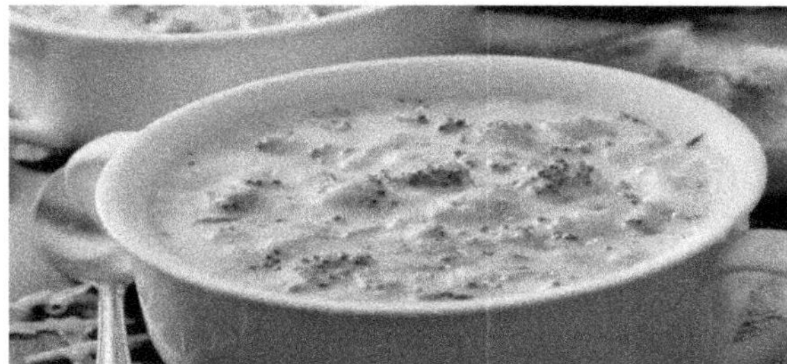

- 4 cups chopped broccoli
- One small onion, chopped two garlic cloves, minced
- 2 cups chicken or veggie broth
- ½ cup unsweetened almond milk
- ¼ cup grated Parmesan cheese
- Salt and pepper to taste
- **Optional toppings:** chopped almonds or chives

Instructions:

1. In a large saucepan, sauté the onion and garlic in olive oil until tender.
2. Add the chopped broccoli and chicken or vegetable broth to the saucepan. Bring to a boil, then decrease the heat and simmer for 10-15 minutes or until the broccoli is cooked.

3. Using an immersion blender or transferring to a blender, mix the soup until smooth.

4. Stir in the almond milk and Parmesan cheese, and season with salt and pepper to taste.
5. Serve hot with optional garnishes of chopped almonds or chives.

This soup is a fantastic alternative for a warm and cozy dinner that's low in carbs and strong in fiber and minerals. Broccoli is a cruciferous vegetable that's abundant in antioxidants, vitamins, and fiber. The almond milk and Parmesan cheese enhance richness and taste without adding additional calories or dairy.

Chicken and Vegetable Stew

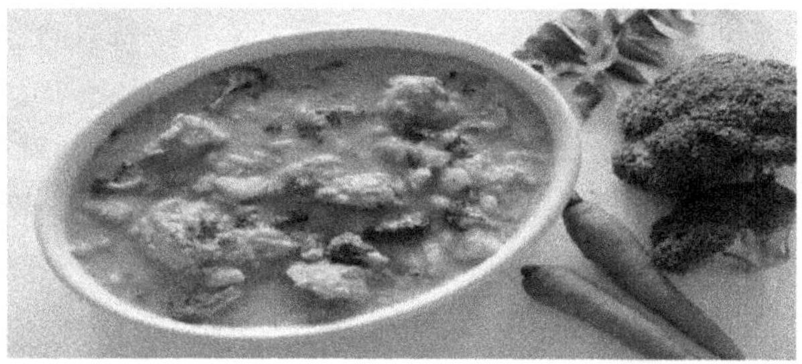

Ingredients:

- One lb. boneless, skinless chicken breasts, cubed one onion, chopped two garlic cloves, minced 2 cups chopped mixed veggies (such as carrots, celery, and bell peppers)
- 2 cups chicken broth
- One can (14 oz.) of chopped tomatoes, drained
- 1 tsp. dried oregano
- 1 tsp. dried basil
- Salt and pepper to taste

Instructions:

1. In a large saucepan, sauté the onion and garlic in a touch of olive oil until tender.

2. Add the cubed chicken and chopped mixed veggies to the saucepan. Cook for 5-7 minutes or until the chicken is browned.

3. Add the chicken stock, diced tomatoes, dried oregano, dry basil, salt, and pepper to the saucepan. Bring to a boil, then decrease the heat and simmer for 20-25 minutes or until the veggies are soft and the chicken is cooked.

4. Serve hot, and enjoy!

This stew is a substantial and healthy dinner that's strong in protein and veggies. The chicken delivers lean protein, while the mixed veggies supply vitamins, minerals, and fiber. You may also add different herbs or spices according to your tastes.

CHAPTER FIVE

Dinner Recipes

Here are two PCOS-friendly supper dishes that are both quick to make and rich in nutrients:

Baked Salmon with Roasted Vegetables

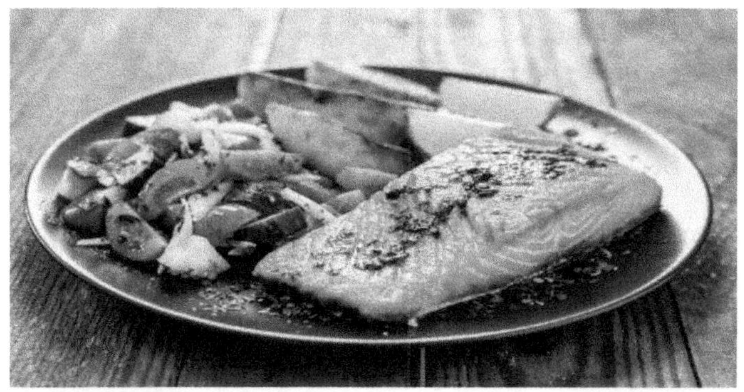

Ingredients:

- Four salmon fillets
- 2 cups mixed veggies (such as broccoli, carrots, and bell peppers)
- 1 tbsp. olive oil
- ½ tsp. garlic powder
- Salt and pepper to taste

Instructions:

1. Preheat the oven to 400°F.

2. Place the salmon fillets on a baking pan lined with parchment paper. Season with salt and pepper.

3. Combine the mixed veggies with olive oil, garlic powder, salt, and pepper in a bowl. Spread the veggies around the salmon fillets on the baking sheet.

4. Bake for 15-20 minutes or until the salmon is cooked and the veggies are soft.

5. Serve hot, and enjoy!

This meal is a terrific alternative for a fast and simple supper that's strong in omega-3 fatty acids, lean protein, and fiber. Salmon is a fatty fish high in omega-3s, while mixed veggies give a range of minerals and fiber.

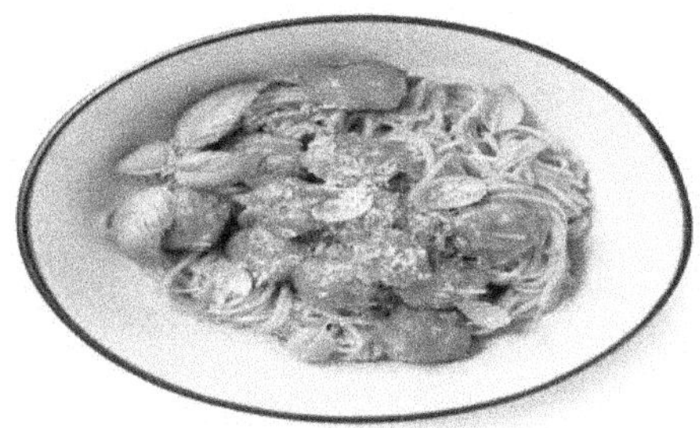

Ingredients:

- One spaghetti squash, halved and seeds removed
- 1 pound. ground turkey, one small onion, and diced
- Two garlic cloves minced
- One egg
- ¼ cup almond flour
- 1 tbsp. dried oregano
- 1 tbsp. dried basil
- One can (14 oz.) of chopped tomatoes, drained
- Salt and pepper to taste

Instructions:

1. Preheat the oven to 400°F.

2. Place the spaghetti squash halves cut side down on a baking sheet. Bake for 30-40 minutes or until the squash is soft.

3. Mix the ground turkey, diced onion, minced garlic, egg, almond flour, dried oregano, dried basil, salt, and pepper in a bowl. Mix thoroughly and shape into meatballs.

4. In a large skillet, fry the meatballs over medium heat for 5-7 minutes or until cooked through.

5. Add the diced tomatoes to the skillet with the meatballs and boil for 5-10 minutes.

6. Using a fork, scrape the spaghetti squash flesh into spaghetti-like strands.

7. Serve the meatballs and tomato sauce over the spaghetti squash strands, and enjoy!

This meal is a nutritious and fulfilling alternative to typical spaghetti and meatballs that are low in carbs and rich in fiber and protein. Spaghetti squash is a healthy food that's fiber and low in calories, while turkey meatballs give lean protein and taste without additional saturated fat.

PCOS-friendly meal ideas

Grilled Chicken with Roasted Vegetables:

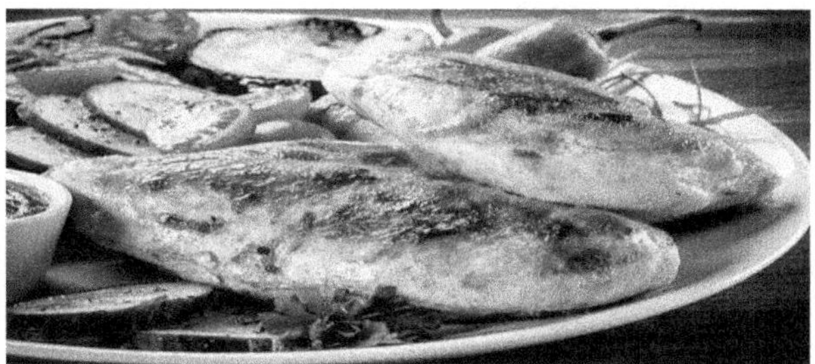

Ingredients:

- Four chicken breasts
- One red bell pepper
- One yellow bell pepper
- One zucchini
- One yellow squash, one red onion
- 2 tbsp olive oil
- 2 tsp dried basil
- 2 tsp dried oregano
- Salt and pepper to taste

Instructions:

1. Preheat the grill to medium-high heat.

2. Cut the bell peppers, zucchini, yellow squash, and red onion into big bite-sized pieces.

3. Combine olive oil, dried basil, dried oregano, salt, and pepper in a dish.

4. Toss the veggies in the oil and herb mixture until coated.

5. Grill the chicken breasts on each side for 6-7 minutes or until cooked through.

6. Place the seasoned veggies on a baking sheet and roast them in the oven at 375°F for 15-20 minutes or until tender.

7. Serve the grilled chicken with the roasted veggies on the side.

This recipe is rich in fiber, vitamins, and protein, making it a perfect choice for a PCOS-friendly supper. You may also change out the veggies or use a different kind of protein depending on your tastes.

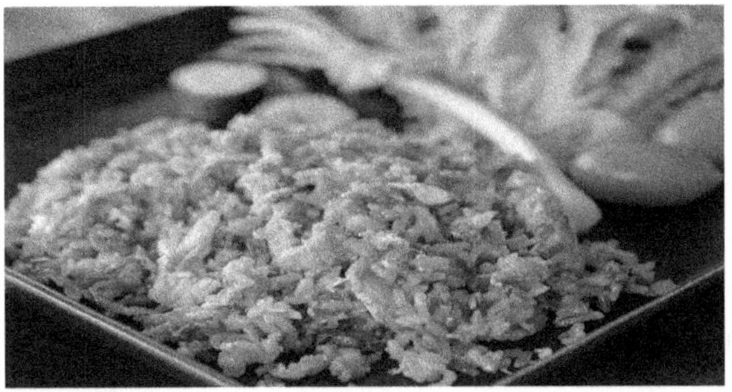

Ingredients:

- 1 cup brown rice
- 2 tbsp vegetable oil
- 1 pound boneless, skinless chicken breast cut into tiny pieces
- One red bell pepper, sliced
- One yellow bell pepper, sliced
- 1 cup snow peas
- 1 cup broccoli florets
- Two cloves garlic, minced
- 1 tsp grated ginger
- 3 tbsp low-sodium soy sauce
- 1 tbsp cornstarch
- 1 tbsp honey
- Salt and pepper to taste
- Chopped green onions for garnish

Instructions:

1. Cook the brown rice according to the package directions and put it aside.
2. Heat the vegetable oil in a large pan over medium-high heat.

3. Add the chicken and stir-fry until browned and cooked, approximately 5-6 minutes.

4. Add the sliced bell peppers, snow peas, broccoli florets, garlic, and ginger to the pan and stir-fry for 3-4 minutes until the veggies are somewhat soft.

5. Whisk together soy sauce, cornstarch, honey, salt, and pepper in a small bowl.

6. Pour the soy sauce mixture into the pan and stir-fry for 2-3 minutes or until the sauce thickens and covers the veggies and chicken.

7. Serve the stir-fry over the cooked brown rice and top with chopped green onions.

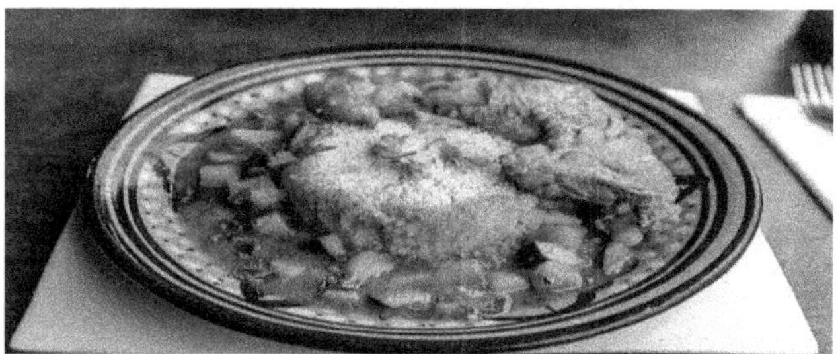

Ingredients:

- Two medium sweet potatoes, peeled and chopped
- One can of black beans, washed and drained
- 1 cup corn kernels
- One red bell pepper, chopped
- One small onion, chopped
- One tablespoon of olive oil
- One teaspoon of ground cumin
- One teaspoon of chili powder
- ½ teaspoon garlic powder
- Salt & pepper, to taste
- Ten corn tortillas
- 2 cups enchilada sauce
- 1 cup shredded cheddar cheese

Instructions:

1. Preheat the oven to 375°F.

2. In a large pan, heat the olive oil over medium-high heat. Add the sweet potatoes, onion, bell pepper, and sauté for 5-7 minutes, or until the veggies are soft.

3. Add the black beans, corn, cumin, chili powder, garlic powder, salt, and pepper to the pan. Cook for another 2-3 minutes or until heated through.

4. Spoon a tiny quantity of enchilada sauce onto the bottom of a 9x13-inch baking dish.

5. Spoon the sweet potato and black bean mixture onto each tortilla and wrap it up firmly. Place the rolled tortillas seam-side down in the baking dish.

6. Pour the leftover enchilada sauce over the tortillas and sprinkle with shredded cheese.

7. Bake for 25-30 minutes or until the enchiladas are hot and bubbling.

8. Serve hot with extra toppings like avocado, sour cream, or chopped cilantro.

This meal is a terrific alternative for a PCOS-friendly supper since it contains fiber, protein, and healthy carbs. Sweet potatoes give a lot of vitamin A and antioxidants, while black beans supply plant-based protein and fiber.

Plus, the enchilada sauce adds a delicious Mexican-inspired flavor to the dish.

Zucchini Noodle and Turkey Meatball Bowl

Ingredients:

- 1 pound ground turkey
- ¼ cup almond flour
- ¼ cup grated Parmesan cheese 1/4 cup chopped fresh parsley
- One egg, two cloves of garlic, and minced
- Salt & pepper, to taste
- Two medium zucchini, spiralized or julienned into noodles
- ½ cup cherry tomatoes, halved
- ½ cup chopped mushrooms
- ¼ cup chopped red onion
- Two tablespoons of olive oil
- Lemon wedges for serving

Instructions:

1. Preheat the oven to 375°F.

2. Combine the ground turkey, almond flour, Parmesan cheese, parsley, egg, garlic, salt, and pepper in a large mixing bowl. Mix thoroughly.

3. Roll the turkey mixture into tiny meatballs approximately 1 inch in diameter.

4. Place the meatballs on a baking sheet lined with parchment paper and bake for 15-20 minutes or until cooked.

5. While the meatballs are cooking, heat the olive oil in a large skillet over medium heat. Add the zucchini noodles, cherry tomatoes, mushrooms, and red onion. Sauté for 5-7 minutes or until the veggies are soft.

6. Divide the zucchini noodle mixture into two bowls.

7. Top each bowl with the cooked meatballs.

8. Serve hot with lemon wedges on the side for squeezing over the top.

This meal is a terrific alternative for a PCOS-friendly supper since it is low in carbs and strong in protein and healthy fats. The zucchini noodles give a low-carb alternative to classic pasta, while the turkey meatballs provide a lean source of protein. The vegetables add vitamins, minerals, and fiber to the dish.

Cauliflower Fried Rice

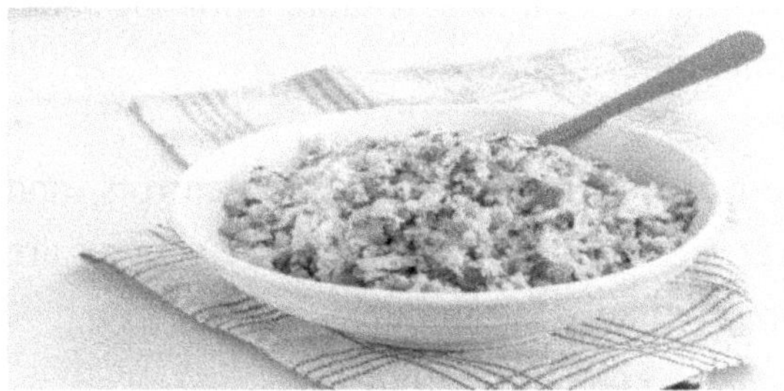

Ingredients:

- One head of cauliflower, riced
- One tablespoon of avocado oil
- Two cloves garlic, minced 1/2 onion, chopped 1/2 cup frozen peas and carrots, thawed two eggs, softly beaten two tablespoons soy sauce or coconut aminos
- Salt & pepper, to taste
- **Optional:** chopped chicken or shrimp, sliced mushrooms, diced bell pepper

Instructions:

1. To rice the cauliflower, chop it into florets and pulse it in a food processor until it resembles rice. Alternatively, you can grate the cauliflower on a box grater.

2. In a large pan, heat the avocado oil over medium heat. Add garlic, onion, and sauté until softened, approximately 2-3 minutes.

3. Add the riced cauliflower, peas and carrots, and other preferred veggies. Cook until the veggies are soft, approximately 5-7 minutes.

4. Push the cauliflower mixture to one side of the pan and pour the beaten eggs into the other. Scramble the eggs until done, then add them to the cauliflower mixture.

5. Add the soy sauce or coconut aminos and whisk to mix. Season with salt and pepper to taste.

6. **Optional:** Add diced chicken or shrimp and sauté until cooked thoroughly.

7. Serve hot as a main meal or side dish.

This dish is a terrific alternative to typical fried rice, which is generally rich in carbs and poor in nutrition. Cauliflower is a low-carb and nutrient-dense replacement for rice and is strong in fiber and antioxidants. This meal is also customizable with extra veggies and protein sources.

CHAPTER SIX

Snack & Appetizer Recipes

Here are some PCOS-friendly snack and appetizer ideas:

Roasted Chickpeas:

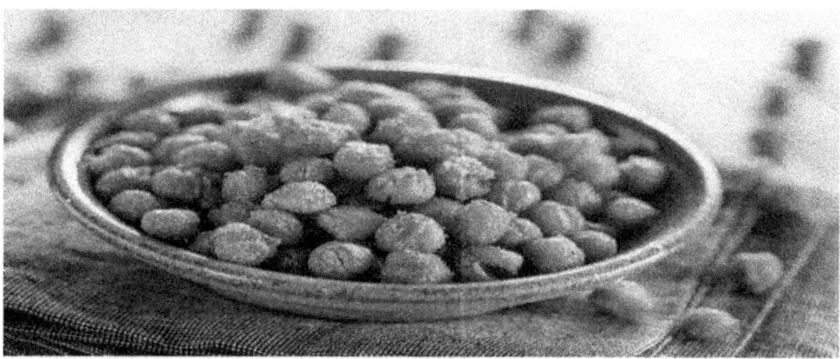

Ingredients:

- One can of chickpeas, drained and rinsed
- One tablespoon of olive oil
- One teaspoon paprika
- One teaspoon cumin
- Salt & pepper, to taste

Instructions:

1. Preheat the oven to 400°F (200°C)

2. Pat the chickpeas dry with a paper towel.

3. Combine chickpeas with olive oil, paprika, cumin, salt, and pepper in a bowl.

4. Spread the chickpeas on a baking sheet and bake for 20-25 minutes or until crispy.

Vegetable Crudité with Hummus:

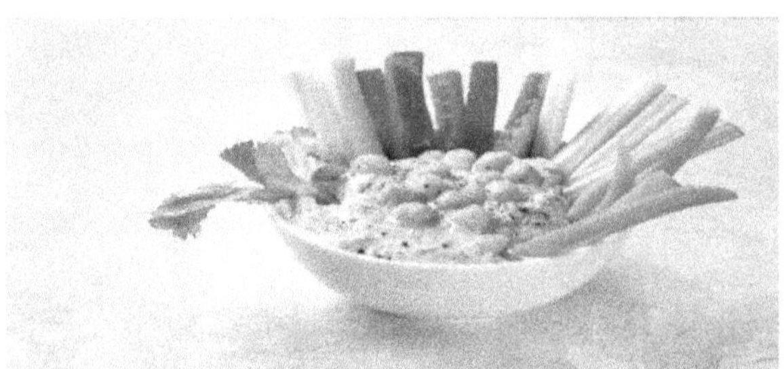

Ingredients:

- Assorted veggies (e.g., carrots, celery, bell peppers, cucumber)
- 1 cup hummus

Instructions:

1. Wash and slice the veggies into bite-sized pieces.

2. Serve with hummus for dipping

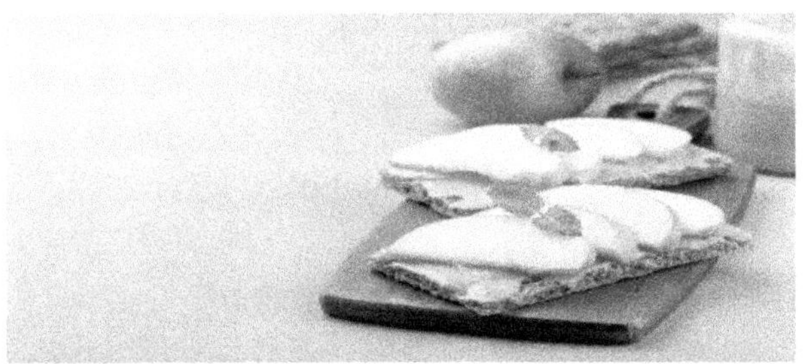

Ingredients:

- One apple, sliced two tablespoons of almond butter

Instructions:

1. Wash and slice the apple.

2. Spread almond butter on each piece and enjoy.

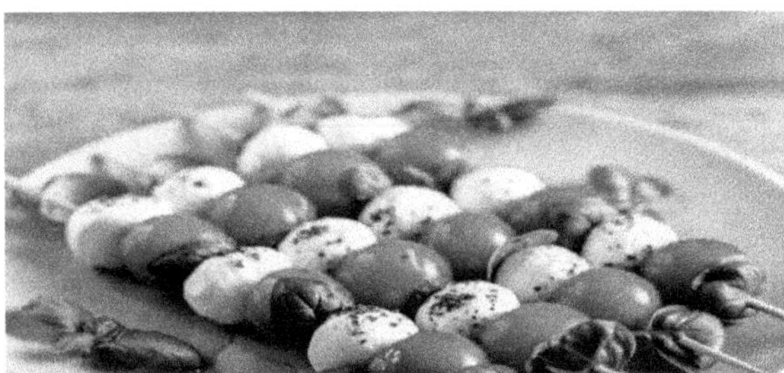

Ingredients:

- Cherry tomatoes
- Fresh basil leaves

* Mozzarella cheese
* Balsamic vinegar for drizzling

Instructions:

1. Wash the cherry tomatoes and basil leaves.

2. Cut the mozzarella cheese into tiny pieces.

3. Thread a cherry tomato, basil leaf, and mozzarella cube onto a skewer.

4. Drizzle with balsamic vinegar.

Greek yogurt with fruit

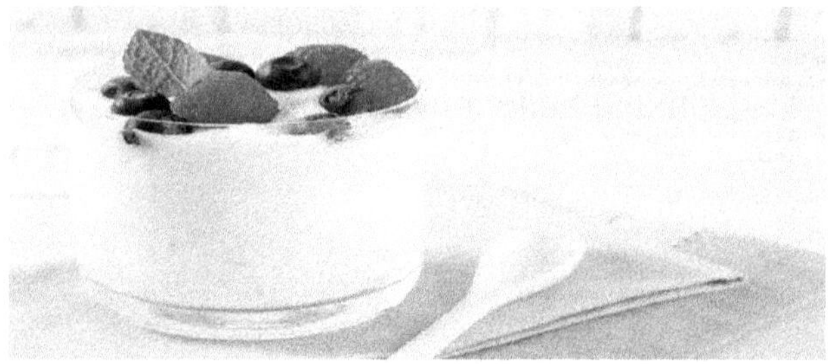

Ingredients:

* 1 cup of plain Greek yogurt
* ½ cup of mixed berries (such as strawberries, blueberries, and raspberries)
* **Optional:** 1 tablespoon of nuts or seeds (such as almonds, walnuts, or chia seeds)

Instructions:

1. Spoon the Greek yogurt into a bowl or serving plate.

2. Rinse the berries and chop any big berries into smaller pieces, if desired.

3. Top the Greek yogurt with the mixed berries.
4. Sprinkle with nuts or seeds if using.

5. Serve and enjoy!

Raw vegetables with hummus

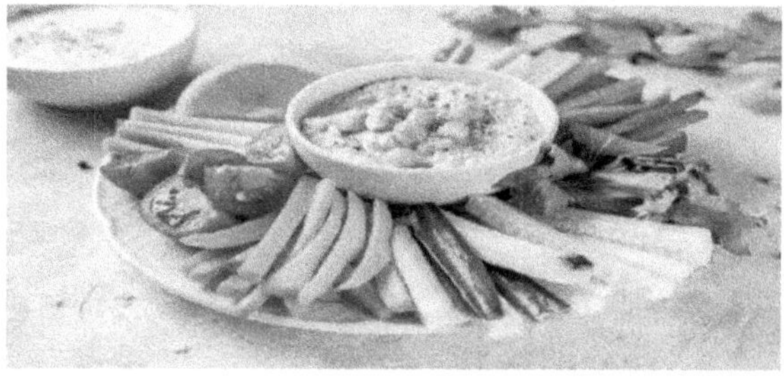

Ingredients:

- 1 cup of your favorite raw vegetables, such as carrots, cucumbers, bell peppers, and celery
- ½ cup of hummus
- **Optional:** herbs and spices, such as parsley, paprika, or cumin

Instructions:

1. Wash and prepare the raw vegetables by slicing them into bite-sized pieces.
2. Spoon the hummus into a small serving plate.
3. Arrange the raw vegetables around the plate of hummus.
4. Sprinkle herbs and spices on top of the hummus, if preferred.

Smoothie

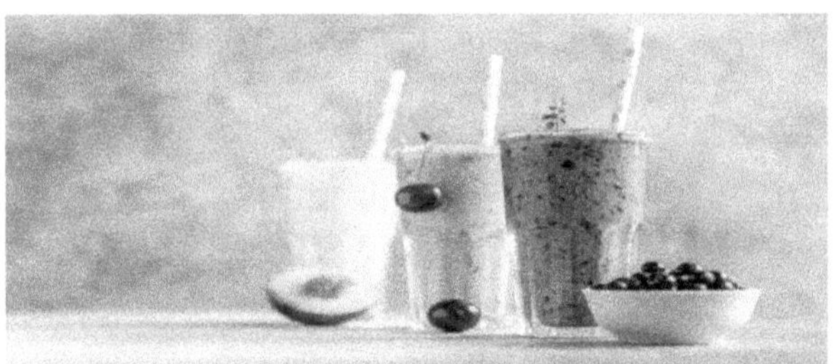

Ingredients:

- 1 cup of frozen mixed berries (such as strawberries, blueberries, and raspberries)
- One banana, peeled and sliced
- 1 cup of unsweetened almond milk (or other non-dairy milk)
- One tablespoon of chia seeds
- **Optional:** Honey or maple syrup for extra sweetness

Instructions:

1. Add the frozen berries, sliced banana, almond milk, and chia seeds to a blender.
2. Blend on high speed until the components are smooth and fully incorporated.

3. Flavor the smoothie and add honey or maple syrup if you like a sweeter flavor.

4. Pour the smoothie into a glass and serve immediately.

CHAPTER SEVEN

Dessert Recipes

Chocolate Avocado Mousse

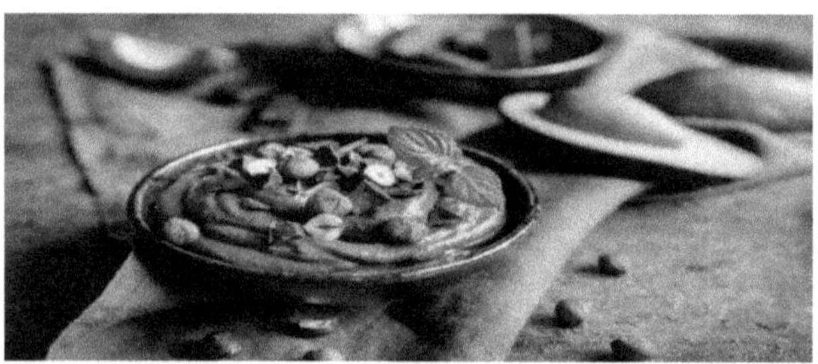

Ingredients:

- Two ripe avocados
- 1/4 cup of unsweetened cocoa powder
- 1/4 cup of almond milk (or other non-dairy milk)
- One teaspoon of vanilla essence
- Two teaspoons of honey or maple syrup

Instructions:

1. Cut the avocados in half and remove the pits.

2. Scoop the avocado flesh into a blender or food processor.

3. Add the cocoa powder, almond milk, vanilla extract, and honey or maple syrup to the blender.

4. Blend on high speed until the components are smooth and fully incorporated.

5. Spoon the mousse into individual serving plates and chill for at least 1 hour before serving.

Berry and Coconut Milk Popsicles

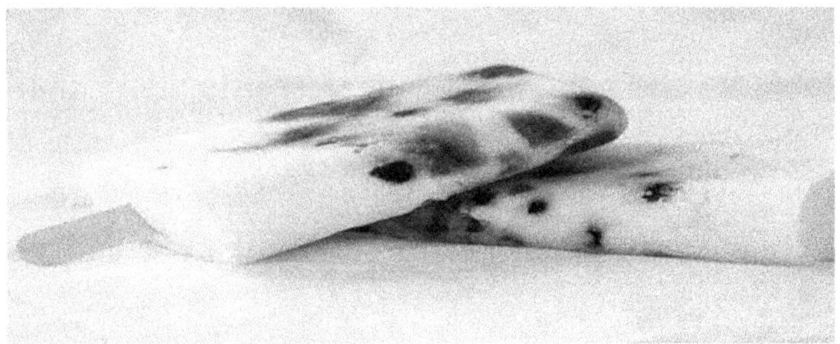

Ingredients:

- 1 cup of mixed berries (such as strawberries, raspberries, and blueberries)
- One can of coconut milk
- One tablespoon of honey or maple syrup

Instructions:

1. Wash and prepare the mixed berries.

2. Divide the berries equally among six popsicle molds.

3. In a blender, mix the coconut milk and honey or maple syrup.

4. Blend on high speed until the contents are fully incorporated.

5. Pour the coconut milk mixture over the fruit in the popsicle molds.

6. Insert popsicle sticks into the molds.

7. Freeze the popsicles for at least 4 hours or until they are frozen.

8. Remove the popsicles from the molds and serve.

Baked Apples with Cinnamon and Almonds

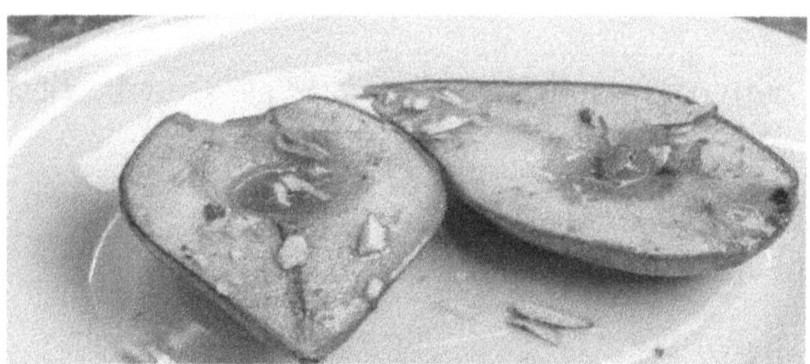

Ingredients:

- Four medium-sized apples
- ¼ cup of chopped almonds
- One tablespoon of cinnamon

- One tablespoon of honey or maple syrup

Instructions:

1. Preheat your oven to 375°F (190°C).

2. Wash and core the apples.

3. Mix the chopped almonds, cinnamon, and honey or maple syrup in a small dish.

4. Stuff the almond mixture into the middle of each apple.

5. Place the filled apples on a baking sheet.

6. Bake the apples for 25-30 minutes or until soft and gently browned.

7. Remove the apples from the oven and allow them cool for a few minutes before serving.

Almond Flour Banana Bread

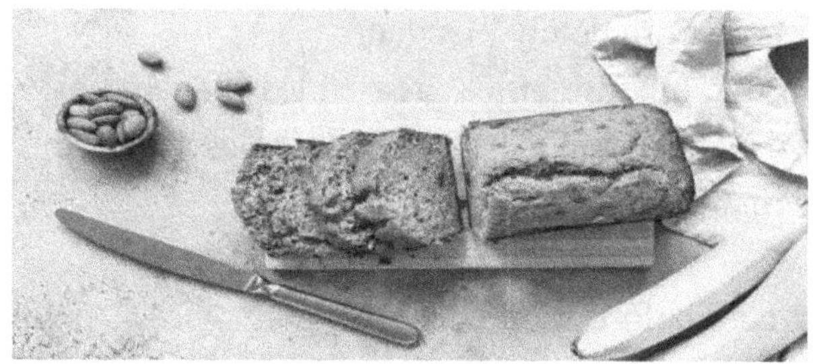

Ingredients:

- 2 cups almond flour
- Two ripe bananas, mashed
- Three eggs
- 1 tsp vanilla extract
- 1 tsp baking soda
- ½ tsp ground cinnamon
- Pinch of salt
- ¼ cup honey
- ¼ cup coconut oil

Instructions:

1. Preheat the oven to 350°F.

2. Mix almond flour, baking soda, cinnamon, and salt.

3. Whisk together bananas, eggs, vanilla extract, honey, and coconut oil in a separate dish.

4. Add the dry ingredients to the wet components and stir until completely blended.

5. Pour the mixture into a greased loaf pan and bake for 45-50 minutes, or until a toothpick inserted in the middle comes out clean.

6. Let cool before slicing and serving.

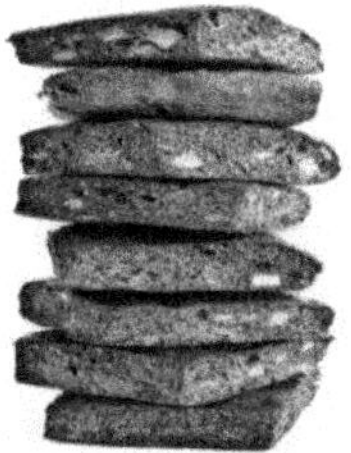

Ingredients:

- Two ripe avocados
- ½ cup honey
- ½ cup unsweetened cocoa powder
- Two eggs
- 1 tsp vanilla extract
- ½ cup almond flour
- ½ tsp baking powder
- Pinch of salt

Instructions:

1. Preheat the oven to 350°F and prepare an 8-inch square baking dish with parchment paper.

2. In a blender or food processor, puree the avocados until smooth.

3. Add honey, cocoa powder, eggs, and vanilla extract to the mixer and process until fully blended.

4. Add almond flour, baking powder, and salt to the blender and mix until blended.

5. Pour the mixture into the prepared baking dish and bake for 25-30 minutes, or until a toothpick inserted in the middle comes out clean.

6. Let cool before slicing and serving.

Oatmeal Raisin Cookies

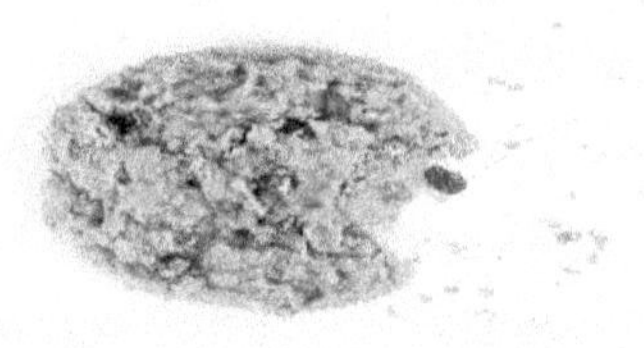

Ingredients:

- 1 cup rolled oats
- ½ cup almond flour
- ½ cup raisins
- ¼ cup honey

- ¼ cup coconut oil
- One egg
- 1 tsp vanilla extract
- 1 tsp ground cinnamon
- 1/2 tsp baking soda
- Pinch of salt

Instructions:

1. Preheat the oven to 350°F and prepare a baking sheet with parchment paper.
2. Whisk together oats, almond flour, raisins, cinnamon, baking soda, and salt in a large basin.

3. Mix honey, coconut oil, egg, and vanilla extract in a separate dish.

4. Add the wet ingredients to the dry ingredients and stir until thoroughly blended.

5. Drop spoonfuls of batter onto the prepared baking sheet and flatten with a fork.

6. Bake for 12-15 minutes or until gently browned.

7. Let cool before serving.

Ingredients:

- One can full-fat coconut milk
- 2 cups mixed berries (fresh or frozen)
- 1 tsp vanilla extract
- 2 tbsp honey (optional)

Instructions:

1. Add all ingredients to a blender and mix until smooth.

2. Pour mixture into popsicle molds and freeze for at least 4 hours.

3. Run them under warm water for a few seconds to remove popsicles from the molds.

CHAPTER EIGHT

PCOS Meal Plans

Here's an example 3-day diet plan for PCOS:

Day 1

- **Breakfast:** Greek yogurt with fruit and nuts/seeds
- **Lunch:** Turkey and avocado lettuce wraps with a side of raw carrots and hummus
- **Dinner:** Grilled chicken with roasted veggies (e.g., bell peppers, zucchini, onions) with a side of quinoa
- **Snack:** Apple slices with almond butter

Day 2

- **Breakfast:** Quinoa breakfast bowl with sautéed spinach, cherry tomatoes, and a fried egg
- **Lunch:** Tuna and white bean salad with mixed greens and a balsamic vinaigrette dressing
- **Dinner:** Zucchini noodle and turkey meatball dish with a side of roasted sweet potato wedges
- **Snack:** Carrot sticks with tzatziki sauce

Day 3

- **Breakfast:** Chia seed pudding with sliced banana and a sprinkle of honey
- **Lunch:** Sweet potato and black bean chili with a side of brown rice
- **Dinner:** Cauliflower fried rice with shrimp and assorted vegetables (e.g., carrots, peas, onions)
- **Snack:** Coconut berry popsicles

Note: This is just an example meal plan and may not be suited for everyone. Engaging with a certified dietitian is crucial to design a tailored meal plan that suits your particular requirements and interests

Sample meal plans for varied nutritional requirements

Sample Meal Plan for Vegetarians

- **Breakfast:** Greek yogurt with berries and nuts/seeds or Veggie Omelet
- **Snack:** Raw vegetables with hummus
- **Lunch:** Quinoa and roasted veggie salad or Sweet Potato and Black Bean Chili
- **Snack:** Apple slices with almond butter
- **Dinner:** Cauliflower Fried Rice or Zucchini Noodles and Turkey Meatball Bowl

Sample Meal Plan for Vegans

- **Breakfast:** Smoothie bowl or Chia Seed Pudding
- **Snack:** Fresh fruit salad
- **Lunch:** Tofu and Vegetable Stir-Fry with Brown Rice or Lentil and Sweet Potato Stew
- **Snack:** Raw vegetables with roasted red pepper hummus
- **Dinner:** Stuffed Portobello Mushrooms or Vegan Butternut Squash Soup

Sample Meal Plan for Gluten-Free

- **Breakfast:** Overnight oats or Quinoa Breakfast Bowl
- **Snack:** Rice cake with almond butter and banana
- **Lunch:** Greek Salad with Grilled Chicken or Grilled Salmon and Vegetable Skewers
- **Snack:** Carrot sticks with roasted garlic hummus
- **Dinner:** Grilled Chicken with Roasted Vegetables or Turkey and Avocado Lettuce Wraps

Sample Meal Plan for Low-Carb

- **Breakfast:** Spinach and Mushroom Omelet or Greek Yogurt with Berries and Nuts/Seeds

- **Snack:** Hard-boiled egg
- **Lunch:** Grilled Chicken Caesar Salad or Turkey and Avocado Lettuce Wraps
- **Snack:** Celery sticks with almond butter
- **Dinner:** Grilled Steak with Asparagus or Baked Salmon with Broccoli

Sample Meal Plan for Keto

- **Breakfast:** Keto Green Smoothie or Bacon and Eggs
- **Snack:** Macadamia nuts
- **Lunch:** Grilled Chicken Caesar Salad or Keto Zucchini Noodles with Meatballs
- **Snack:** Cheese cubes
- **Dinner:** Keto Meatloaf with Mashed Cauliflower or Grilled Steak with Asparagus

How to tailor meal plans for your requirements

To modify meal plans for your requirements, follow these steps:

1. **Determine your caloric needs:** The quantity of calories you require each day relies on different parameters, including age, gender, weight, height,

and activity level. You may use an online calculator to calculate your daily calorie requirements.

2. **Determine your macronutrient needs:** Macronutrients are carbs, proteins, and lipids. The proportion of macronutrients you need to take in your diet depends on your requirements and preferences. Generally, a balanced PCOS-friendly diet comprises roughly 50% carbs, 20-25% protein, and 25-30% healthy fats.

3. **Identify your dietary preferences and allergies:** List items you love eating and any food sensitivities you may have. This will help you build a food plan that is both fun and safe for you to consume.

4. **Plan your meals:** Pick items corresponding to your calorie and macronutrient demands and dietary preferences. For example, if you require 1500 calories daily, plan three meals containing approximately 500 calories, plus two snacks with roughly 100-150 calories each. Also, try cooking meals in advance to save time throughout the week.

5. **Review your success:** After following your food plan for a few weeks, review your progress by noting any changes in your weight, energy levels, and symptoms. If you discover that you need to tweak your meal plan to meet your requirements better, make the required modifications and continue tracking your progress.

CHAPTER TEN

Living with PCOS

Living with PCOS may be tough, but there are strategies to reduce symptoms and enhance the quality of life. Here are some tips for living with PCOS:

1. **Stay active:** Regular exercise can help improve insulin resistance, reduce inflammation, and maintain a healthy weight. Aim for at least 150 minutes of moderate-intensity exercise per week.

2. **Get adequate sleep:** Lack of sleep may raise insulin resistance and cortisol levels, aggravating PCOS symptoms. Aim for 7-9 hours of sleep per night.

3. **Manage stress:** Stress may increase PCOS symptoms, so finding techniques to manage stress is vital. This may involve practicing relaxation methods like deep breathing, meditation, or yoga.

4. **Stay hydrated:** Drinking enough water can help manage weight and reduce bloating. Aim for at least 8 cups of water per day.

5. **Keep track of your menstrual cycle:** Keeping a note of your menstrual cycle might help you discover anomalies and monitor progress over time. This might also be useful when discussing treatment alternatives with your healthcare physician.

6. **Seek support:** Living with PCOS can be challenging, and having a support system can be helpful. This can include family, friends, support groups, and online communities.

7. **Follow a PCOS-friendly diet:** Eating a balanced diet emphasizing healthy foods will help control PCOS symptoms. Focus on meals that are low in added sugars, saturated fats, and refined carbs, and instead pick foods rich in fiber, protein, and healthy fats.

Remember, PCOS is a chronic illness that needs continuing care. Engaging with your healthcare physician is vital to build a specific treatment plan that works for you.

Lifestyle suggestions for controlling PCOS

Here are some lifestyle tips that may help manage PCOS:

1. **Maintain a healthy weight:** Losing even a minor amount of weight will help control PCOS symptoms.

2. **Regular exercise:** may help increase insulin sensitivity, reduce blood sugar levels, and control weight.

3. **Follow a healthy diet:** Eating a balanced and nutritious diet might help control PCOS symptoms. Incorporate foods that are low in glycemic index, high in fiber, and rich in nutrients.

4. **Manage stress:** Stress may influence hormone levels and increase PCOS symptoms. Engage in stress-reducing activities like yoga, meditation, or deep breathing techniques.

5. **Get adequate sleep:** Poor sleep may exacerbate insulin resistance and promote inflammation, aggravating PCOS symptoms.

6. **Quit smoking:** Smoking may aggravate insulin resistance and raise the risk of various health issues.

7. **Stay hydrated:** Drinking enough water can help flush out toxins and reduce inflammation.

8. **Consult a healthcare practitioner:** Regular check-ups with a healthcare provider may help control PCOS symptoms and monitor possible health problems.

It is essential to note that these lifestyle guidelines may not work for everyone. Speaking with a healthcare specialist for individualized guidance on controlling PCOS is always encouraged.

Self-care techniques for PCOS

Polycystic Ovary Syndrome (PCOS) may be a tough illness to treat. In addition to medical treatments and dietary adjustments, implementing self-care practices may help reduce symptoms and enhance general well-being. Here are some self-care strategies for PCOS:

1. **Regular exercise**: may help improve insulin resistance, increase weight reduction, and lower stress levels. Aim for at least 30 minutes of moderate-intensity exercise most days of the week.

2. **Get adequate sleep:** Aim for at least 7-8 hours every night to help decrease stress and enhance hormonal balance.

3. **Manage stress:** Chronic stress might increase PCOS symptoms. Engage in stress-reducing activities such as yoga, meditation, or deep breathing techniques.

4. **Prioritize self-care activities:** Make time for things that offer pleasure and relaxation, such as reading, bathing, or in nature.

5. **Connect with others:** PCOS may be lonely, so connecting with those who understand what you're going through is crucial. Join a support group, seek out therapy, or connect with others online.

6. **Practice mindfulness:** Mindfulness techniques like meditation or journaling may help decrease stress and increase emotional well-being.

7. **Take care of your mental health:** PCOS might be connected with an increased risk of sadness and anxiety. Don't hesitate to seek professional assistance if you're dealing with your mental health.

Remember, controlling PCOS is a journey, and it's crucial to emphasize self-care along the way.

Additional resources for living with PCOS

There are several resources accessible for persons living with PCOS. Here are a few examples:

1. **PCOS Challenge:** PCOS Challenge is a nonprofit organization committed to increasing awareness of PCOS and providing support and resources for individuals afflicted by the illness. They provide activities and services, including support groups, internet resources, and instructional materials.

2. **National Polycystic Ovary Syndrome Association:** The National Polycystic Ovary Syndrome Association is another nonprofit organization that offers information, support, and advocacy for those with PCOS. They provide some tools, including online support groups, instructional materials, and information on treatment alternatives.

3. **The PCOS Diet Center:** The PCOS Nutrition Center is a website and resource center committed to assisting persons with PCOS manage their symptoms via diet and lifestyle modifications.

They provide various tools, including articles, recipes, and coaching services.

4. **PCOS Awareness Association:** The PCOS Awareness Association is a nonprofit organization that works to enhance awareness of PCOS and improve the lives of individuals afflicted by the disease. They provide some tools, including online support groups, instructional materials, and information on treatment alternatives.

5. **Your healthcare provider:** Your healthcare practitioner is a vital resource for controlling PCOS. They may help you build a tailored treatment plan, give counseling on lifestyle modifications, and refer you to experts if required.

These are just a few examples of the many resources available for people with PCOS. Engaging with your healthcare practitioner and a team of professionals is crucial to establish a thorough treatment plan that suits your particular requirements.